The Ultimate Bread Machine Cooking Guide

Delicious Sweet and Savoury Dough Recipes For Everyone

Jude Lamb

1

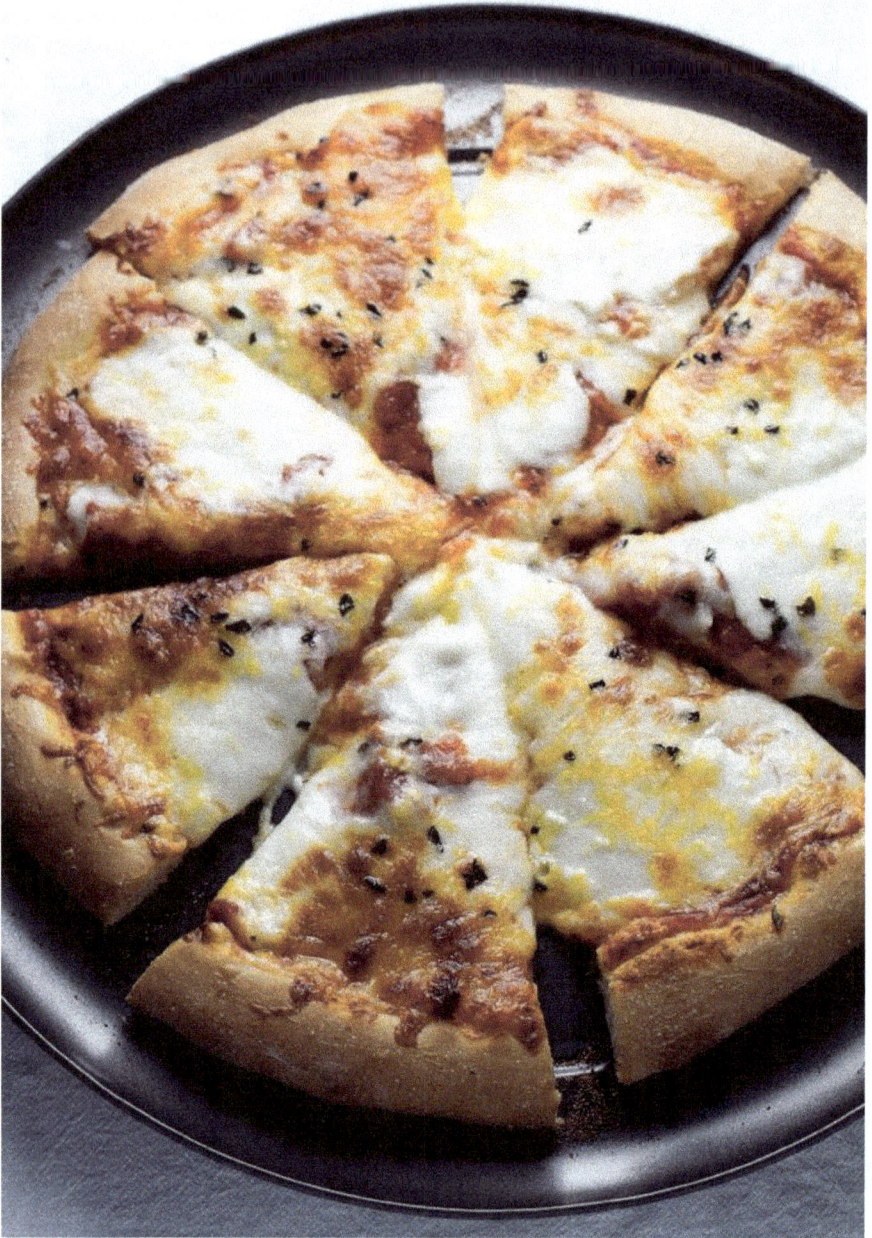

Table of contents

Making Bread

There is nothing like the scent of freshly baked bread to greet you when you wake up. Bakers traditionally produced their products during the early hours meaning their loaves were fresh, hot, and mouth-watering tasty for hungry customers wanting a slice of bread to go with a slap-up breakfast.

Bread historically dates back to Neolithic or even prehistoric times in its earliest incarnation.

Prime ingredients include flour and water used to make the dough. The dough can have numerous additives to offer assorted consistency, flavors, and healthy preferences. Additives may include yeast, fat, salt, baking soda, fruits, spices, eggs, milk, sugar, or vegetables. You can even add seeds to the bread, oils, and nuts. Bread is quite a versatile product and can be devoured on its own or as an accompaniment to the main dish. The dough is traditionally baked, but modern alternatives could include steaming.

The outer part of the bread, commonly known as the crust, can be baked into a hard or soft version. The inner part of the bread is classed as the "crumb," strangely not the small bits that cover your lap.

The prime time to eat a loaf of bread is soon after it has been removed from the oven. At this delicious time, the bread is warm, aromatic, and fresh. Leaving the bread for any length of time will cause the bread to become stale.

A quirk dating back to the 13th century was the Baker's Dozen.

A Baker's Dozen, ironic as it was from the 13th century, relates to 13 items making a dozen instead of the usual 1 1/2. As history would have us believe, a Baker's dozen suggested that punishment was administered to bakers who short-changed their customers. One way to ensure that a customer always received a full quota was to give more bread than paid for. Furthermore, if one loaf was damaged, burnt or was of unacceptable quality, there were still 1 1/2 loaves available for the customer.

Another explanation of the Baker's Dozen, and slightly more believable, is that when round loaves were placed on a standard baking tray, the configuration was 3+2+3+2+3 which gave a greater density to the tray and allowed easier stacking.

Over the decades, the baking of bread has followed the path of many traditions updated to reflect the changing needs of society. Whereas bread was always the preserve of the local baker, modern supermarkets now have their own "in-house" ovens, and bread is baked to suit customer demand.

Orange Bread

Preparation Time: 15 minutes
1½-Pound Loaf

Ingredients:

- ☐ 1¼ cups water
- ☐ 3 tablespoons powdered milk
- ☐ 1½ tablespoons vegetable oil
- ☐ 3 tablespoons honey
- ☐ 2½ cups bread flour
- ☐ ¾ cup amaranth flour
- ☐ 1/3 cup whole-wheat flour
- ☐ ¾ teaspoon salt
- ☐ 3 tablespoons fresh orange zest, grated finely
- ☐ 2¼ teaspoons active dry yeast

Directions:

1. Place all ingredients in the baking pan of the bread machine in the order recommended by the manufacturer.
2. Place the baking pan in the bread machine and close the lid.
3. Select Basic setting.
4. Press the start button.

5. Carefully, remove the baking pan from the machine and then invert the bread pound onto a wire rack to cool completely before slicing.

6. With a sharp knife, cut bread pound into desired-sized pounds and serve.

Nutrition:

- Calories: 197
- Total Fat: 2.9 g
- Saturated Fat: 0.6 g
- Cholesterol: 0 mg
- Sodium: 182 mg
- Carbohydrates: 36.9 g
- Fiber: 2.6 g
- Sugars: 5.6 g
- Protein: 6.1 g

Banana Chocolate Chip Bread

Preparation Time: 15 minutes
1- Pound Loaf

Ingredients:

- ½ cup warm milk
- 2 eggs
- ½ cup butter, melted
- 1 teaspoon vanilla extract
- 3 medium ripe bananas, peeled and mashed
- 1 cup granulated white sugar
- 2 cups all-purpose flour
- ½ teaspoon salt
- 2 teaspoons baking powder
- 1 teaspoon baking soda
- ½ cup chocolate chips

Directions:

Add ingredients (except for cranberries) in the baking pan of the bread machine in the order recommended by the manufacturer.

Place the baking pan in the bread machine and close the lid.

Select Quick Bread setting.

Press the start button.

Wait for the bread machine to beep before adding the chocolate chips.

Carefully, remove the baking pan from the machine and then invert the bread pound onto a wire rack to cool completely before slicing.

With a sharp knife, cut bread pound into desired-sized pounds and serve.

Nutrition:

- Calories: 215
- Total Fat: 1½ g
- Saturated Fat: 5 g
- Cholesterol: 31½ mg
- Sodium: 125 mg
- Carbohydrates: 33.4 g
- Fiber: 1.2 g
- Sugars: 11 g
- Protein: 3.2 g

Sweet Potato Bread

Preparation Time: 15 minutes

Cooking Time: 3 hours

1-Pound Loaf

Ingredients:

☐ ½ cup warm water

☐ 1 teaspoon pure vanilla extract

☐ 1 cup boiled sweet potato, peeled, and mashed

☐ 4 cups bread flour

☐ ½ teaspoon ground cinnamon

☐ 2 tablespoons butter, softened

☐ 1/3 cup brown sugar

☐ 1 teaspoon salt

☐ 2 teaspoons active dry yeast

☐ 2 tablespoons powdered milk

Directions:

1. Place all ingredients in the baking pan of the bread machine in the order recommended by the manufacturer.

2. Place the baking pan in the bread machine and close the lid.

3. Select White Bread setting.

4. Press the start button.

5. Carefully, remove the baking pan from the machine and then invert the bread pound onto a wire rack to cool completely before slicing.

6. With a sharp knife, cut bread pound into desired-sized pounds and serve.

Nutrition:

- Calories: 195
- Total Fat: 1.1 g
- Saturated Fat: 1 g
- Cholesterol: 4 mg
- Sodium: 249 mg
- Carbohydrates: 30.2 g
- Fiber: 1.4 g
- Sugars: 4.4 g
- Protein: 4.1 g

Gingerbread

Preparation Time: 15 minutes

1½ Pounds Loaf

Ingredients:

- ¾ cup milk
- ¼ cup molasses
- 1 egg
- 3 tablespoons butter
- 31/3 cups bread flour
- 1 tablespoon brown sugar
- ¾ teaspoon salt
- ¾ teaspoon ground cinnamon
- ¾ teaspoon ground ginger
- 2¼ teaspoons active dry yeast
- 1/3 cup raisins

Directions:

1. Place all ingredients (except for raisins) in the baking pan of the bread machine in the order recommended by the manufacturer.
2. Place the baking pan in the bread machine and close the lid.
3. Select Basic setting and then Light Crust.

4. Press the start button.

5. Wait for the bread machine to beep before adding the raisins.

6. Carefully, remove the baking pan from the machine and then invert the bread pound onto a wire rack to cool completely before slicing.

7. With a sharp knife, cut bread pound into desired- sized pounds and serve.

Nutrition:

- Calories: 210
- Total Fat: 4 g
- Saturated Fat: 2.2 g
- Cholesterol: 23 mg
- Sodium: 180 mg
- Carbohydrates: 36 g
- Fiber: 1.3 g
- Sugars: 7.7 g
- Protein: 5 g

Raisin Cinnamon Swirl Bread

Preparation Time: 25 minutes
1½-Pound Loaf

Ingredients:

Dough

- ¼ cup milk
- 1 large egg, beaten
- Water, as required
- ¼ cup butter, softened
- 1/3 cup white sugar
- 1 teaspoon salt
- 3½ cups bread flour
- 2 teaspoons active dry yeast
- ½ cup raisins

Cinnamon Swirl

- 1/3 cup white sugar
- 3 teaspoons ground cinnamon
- 2 egg whites, beaten
- 1/3 cup butter, melted and cooled

Directions:

For bread:

1. Place milk and egg into a small bowl.
2. Add enough water to make 1 cup of mixture.
3. Place the egg mixture into the baking pan of the bread machine.
4. Place the remaining ingredients (except for raisins) on top in the order recommended by the manufacturer.
5. Place the baking pan in the bread machine and close the lid.
6. Select Dough cycle.
7. Press the start button.
8. Wait for the bread machine to beep before adding the raisins.
9. After Dough cycle completes, remove the dough from the bread pan and place it onto lightly floured surface.
10. Roll the dough into a 1¼ x1½ -inch rectangle.

For swirl:

1. Mix together the sugar and cinnamon.
2. Brush the dough rectangle with 1 egg white, followed by the melted butter.
3. Now, sprinkle the dough with cinnamon sugar, leaving about a 1-inch border on each side.
4. From the short side, roll the dough and pinch the ends underneath.
5. Grease pound pan and place the dough.

6. With a kitchen towel, cover the pound pan and place in warm place for 1 hour or until doubled in size.

7. Preheat your oven to 350° F.

8. Brush the top of dough with remaining egg white.

9. Bake for approximately 35 minutes or until a wooden skewer inserted in the center comes out clean.

10. Remove the bread pan and place onto a wire rack to cool for about 15 minutes.

11. Cool bread before slicing

Nutrition:

- Calories: 297
- Total Fat: 11 g
- Saturated Fat: 6.3 g
- Cholesterol: 41 mg
- Sodium: 277 mg
- Carbohydrates: 46.2 g
- Fiber: 1.7 g
- Sugars: 11 g
- Protein: 5.6 g

Chocolate Chip Bread

Preparation Time: 15 minutes

1½-Pound Loaf

Ingredients:

- 1 cup milk
- ¼ cup water
- 1 egg, beaten
- 2 tablespoons butter, softened
- 3 cups bread flour
- 2 tablespoons white sugar
- 1 teaspoon salt
- 1 teaspoon ground cinnamon
- 1½ teaspoons active dry yeast
- ¾ cup semi-sweet mini chocolate chips

Directions:

1. Put ingredients (except the chocolate chips) in the baking pan of the bread machine in the order recommended by the manufacturer.
2. Place the baking pan in the bread machine and close the lid.
3. Select Mix Bread setting.
4. Press the start button.

5. Wait for the bread machine to beep before adding chocolate chips.

6. Carefully, remove the baking pan from the machine and then invert the bread pound onto a wire rack to cool completely before slicing.

7. With a sharp knife, cut bread pound into desired-sized pounds and serve.

Nutrition:

- Calories: 226
- Total Fat: 7 g
- Saturated Fat: 4.1 g
- Cholesterol: 1 mg
- Sodium: 240 mg
- Carbohydrates: 36.2 g
- Fiber: 1.1 g
- Sugars: 5 g
- Protein: 4.6 g

Pizza Dough

Preparation Time: 10 minutes
1-Pound Loaf

Ingredients:

- 1 cup of warm water
- ¾ teaspoon salt
- 2 tablespoons olive oil
- 2½ cups flour
- 2 teaspoons sugar
- 2 teaspoons yeast

Directions:

1. Put ingredients in the bread maker.
2. Enable the Dough program and start the cycle.
3. Put the finished dough in a greased form or pan and distribute it. Allow standing for 5minutes.
4. Preheat the oven to 400°F. On top of the dough, place the pizza sauce and the filling. Top with grated cheese.
5. For 1 to 15 minutes, bake till the edge is browned.

Nutrition:

- Calories: 194
- Total Fat: 15.7 g

- Saturated Fat: 2.3 g
- Cholesterol: 0 mg
- Sodium: 180 mg
- Carbohydrates: 12 g
- Dietary Fiber: 5.1 g
- Sugars: 4.4 g Protein: 17.7 g

Pizza Basis

Preparation Time: 10 minutes
1½-Pound Loaf

Ingredients:

- 1¼ cups warm water
- 2 cups flour
- 1 cup Semolina flour
- ½ teaspoon sugar
- 2 teaspoons salt
- 1 teaspoon olive oil
- 2 teaspoons yeast

Directions:

1. Place all the ingredients in the bread maker's bucket in the order recommended by the manufacturer. Select the Dough program.
2. After the dough has risen, use it as the base for the pizza.

Nutrition:

- Calories: 192
- Total Fat: 4.4g
- Saturated Fat: 0.6g
- Cholesterol: 0mg

- Sodium: 480g
- Carbohydrates: 15.6g
- Dietary Fiber: 5.9g
- Total Sugars: 1.5 g
- Protein: 1.9g

Cinnamon Raisin Buns

Preparation Time: 1 hour
1-Pound Loaf

Ingredients:

For dough

- ½ cup milk
- ½ cup water
- 2 tablespoons butter
- ¾ teaspoon salt
- 3 cups flour
- 2¼ teaspoons yeast
- 3 tablespoons sugar
- 1 egg

For filling

- 3 tablespoons butter, melted
- ¾ teaspoon ground cinnamon
- 1/3 cup sugar
- 1/3 cup raisins
- 1/3 cup chopped walnuts

For glaze

- 1 cup powdered sugar

- 1½ tablespoons melted butter
- ¼ teaspoon vanilla
- 1½ tablespoons milk

Directions:

1. In a saucepan, heat ½ cup of milk, water, and 2 tablespoons of butter until they become hot.

2. Put the milk mixture, salt, flour, yeast, sugar, and eggs in the bread maker's bucket in the order recommended by the manufacturer. Select the Dough program. Click Start.

3. When through with the cycle, take out the dough from the bread maker. On a flour-covered surface, roll the dough into a large rectangle. Lubricate with softened butter.

4. Mix the cinnamon and sugar. Sprinkle the rectangle with the mixture. Generously sprinkle with raisins and/or chopped nuts.

5. Roll the dough into a roll, starting from the long side. Cut into 1½ pieces. Put the buns slit-side down on a greased baking tray (25x35cm).

6. Cover and put in the heat until the dough almost doubles, about 30 minutes.

7. Preheat the oven to 375° F. Mix the powdered sugar, 1½ tablespoon melted butter, vanilla, and 1 ½ tablespoon milk to get a thick frosting set it aside.

8. Bake the buns in a preheated oven for 1 - 25 minutes, until browned. Remove and allow to cool down for 5 minutes. Frost the cooled buns with icing.

Nutrition:

- Calories: 301
- Total Fat: 9.2 g
- Saturated Fat: 4.3 g
- Cholesterol: 31mg
- Sodium: 180 g
- Carbohydrate: 53.2 g
- Dietary Fiber: 1.5 g
- Total Sugars: 27.9 g
- Protein: 5.2 g

Italian Pie Calzone

Preparation Time: 1 hour
1½-Pound Loaf

Ingredients:

- 1¼ cups water
- 1 teaspoon salt
- 3 cups flour
- 1 teaspoon milk powder
- 1½ tablespoons sugar
- 2 teaspoons yeast
- ¾ cup tomato sauce for pizza
- 1¼ cups grated mozzarella
- 2 tablespoons butter, melted

Directions:

- Put water, salt, bread baking flour, soluble milk, sugar, and yeast in the bread maker's bucket in the order recommended by the manufacturer. Select the Dough setting.
- After the end of the cycle, roll the dough on a lightly floured surface; form a rectangle measuring 45 x 25 cm. Transfer to a lightly oiled baking tray.
- In a small bowl, spoon the pizza sauce in a strip along the center of the dough, and add the mozzarella.

- Make diagonal incisions at a distance of 1½ cm from each other at the sides, receding 1½ cm from the filling.
- Cross the strips on top of the filling, moistening it with the water. Lubricate with melted butter.
- For 35 to 45 minutes bake at 360° F

Nutrition:
- Calories: 247
- Total Fat: 9.2 g
- Saturated Fat: 3.9 g
- Cholesterol: 22 mg
- Sodium: 590 g
- Carbohydrates: 32 g
- Dietary Fiber: 1.5 g
- Sugars: 2.1½ g
- Protein: 11 g

Extra Buttery White Bread

Preparation Time: 10 minutes

1½-Pound Loaf

Ingredients:

- 1½ cups milk
- 4 tablespoons unsalted butter
- 3 cups bread flour
- 1½ tablespoons white granulated sugar
- 1½ teaspoons salt
- 1½ teaspoons bread machine yeast

Directions:

1. Soften the butter in your microwave.
2. Add each ingredient to the bread machine in the order and at the temperature recommended by your bread machine manufacturer.
3. Close the lid, select the basic or white bread, medium crust setting on your bread machine, and press start.
4. When the bread machine has finished baking, remove the bread and put it on a cooling rack.

Nutrition:

- Calories: 184

- Sodium: 360 mg
- Carbohydrates: 22 g
- Fat. 1 g
- Protein: 4 g

Mom's White Bread

Preparation Time: 10 minutes

1½-Pound Loaf

Ingredients:

- 1 cup and 3 tablespoons water
- 2 tablespoons vegetable oil
- 1½ teaspoons salt
- 2 tablespoons sugar
- 3¼ cups white bread flour
- 2 teaspoons active dry yeast

Directions:

1. Add each ingredient to the bread machine in the order and at the temperature recommended by your bread machine manufacturer.
2. Close the lid, select the basic or white bread, medium crust setting on your bread machine, and press start.
3. When the bread machine has finished baking, remove the bread and put it on a cooling rack.

Nutrition:

- Calories: 175
- Carbohydrates: 10 g

- Fat: 3 g
- Protein: 90 g
- Sodium: 360 mg

Vegan White Bread

Preparation Time: 10 minutes

2 -Pound Loaf

Ingredients:

- 11/3cups water
- 1/3 cup plant milk (I use silk soy original)
- 1½ teaspoons salt
- 2 tablespoons granulated sugar
- 2 tablespoons vegetable oil
- 3½ cups all-purpose flour
- 1¾ teaspoons bread machine yeast

Directions:

1. Add each ingredient to the bread machine in the order and at the temperature recommended by your bread machine manufacturer.
2. Close the lid, select the basic or white bread, medium crust setting on your bread machine, and press start.
3. When the bread machine has finished baking, remove the bread and put it on a cooling rack.

Nutrition:

- Calories: 175

- Carbohydrates: 13 g
- Fat: 2 g
- Protein: 3 g
- Sodium: 360 mg

Rice Flour Rice Bread

Preparation Time: 15 minutes
2-Pound Loaf

Ingredients:

- 3 eggs
- 1½ cups water
- 3 tablespoons vegetable oil
- 1 teaspoon apple cider vinegar
- 2¼ teaspoons active dry yeast
- 3¼ cups white rice flour
- 2½ teaspoons Xanthan gum
- 1½ teaspoons salt
- ½ cup dry milk powder
- 3 tablespoons white sugar

Directions:

1. In a medium-size bowl, add the oil, water, eggs, and vinegar.
2. In a large dish, add the yeast, salt, Xanthan gum, dry milk powder, rice flour, and sugar. Mix with a whisk until incorporated.

3. Add each ingredient to the bread machine in the order and at the temperature recommended by your bread machine manufacturer.

4. Close the lid, select the whole wheat, medium crust setting on your bread machine, and press start.

5. When the bread machine has finished baking, remove the bread and put it on a cooling rack.

Nutrition:

- Calories: 215
- Carbohydrates: 24 g
- Fat: 1 g
- Protein: 2 g
- Sodium: 360 mg

Italian White Bread

Preparation Time: 10 minutes
1-Pound Loaf

Ingredients:

- ¾ cup cold water
- 2 cups bread flour
- 1 tablespoon sugar
- 1 teaspoon salt
- 1 tablespoon olive oil
- 1 teaspoon active dry yeast

Directions:

1. Add each ingredient to the bread machine in the order and at the temperature recommended by your bread machine manufacturer.
2. Close the lid, select the Italian or basic bread, low crust setting on your bread machine, and press start.
3. When the bread machine has finished baking, remove the bread and put it on a cooling rack.

Nutrition:

- Calories: 171
- Carbohydrates: 11 g

- Fat: 1 g
- Protein: 2 g
- Sodium: 240 mg

Anadama White Bread

Preparation Time: 10 minutes

1½-Pound Loaf

Ingredients:

- 1½ cups warm water
- 1/3 cup molasses
- 1½ tablespoons butter at room temperature
- 1 teaspoon salt
- 1/3 cup yellow cornmeal
- 3½ cups bread flour
- 2½ teaspoons bread machine yeast

Directions:

1. Add each ingredient to the bread machine in the order and at the temperature recommended by your bread machine manufacturer.
2. Close the lid, select the basic bread, low crust setting on your bread machine, and press start.
3. When the bread machine has finished baking, remove the bread and put it on a cooling rack.

Nutrition:

- Calories: 186

- Carbohydrates: 19 g
- Fat: 1 g
- Protein: 2 g
- Sodium: 240 mg

Soft White Bread

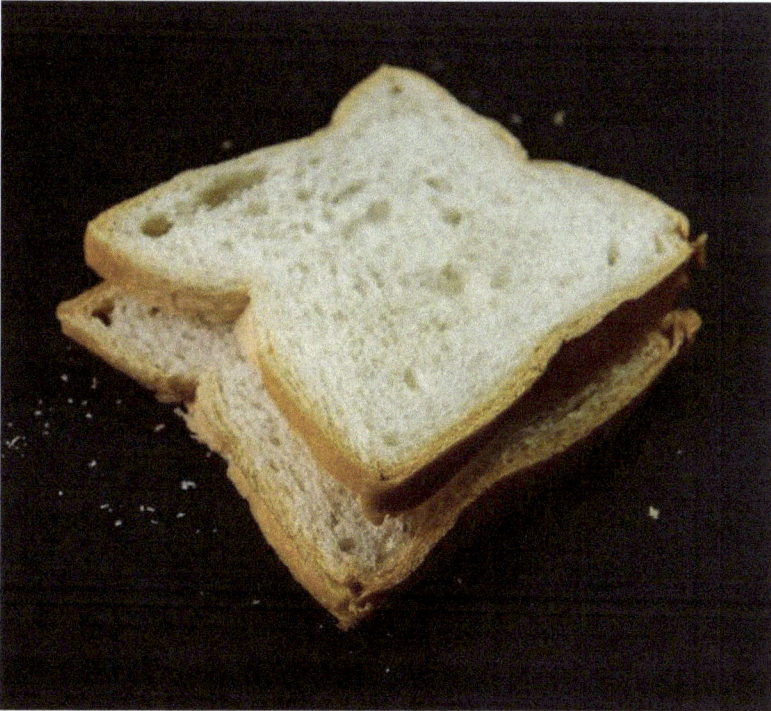

Preparation Time: 10 minutes

2-Pound Loaf

Ingredients:

- 2 cups water
- 4 teaspoons yeast
- 6 tablespoons sugar
- ½ cup vegetable oil

- 2 teaspoons salt
- 3 cups strong white flour

Directions:

1. Add each ingredient to the bread machine in the order and at the temperature recommended by your bread machine manufacturer.
2. Close the lid, select the basic bread, low crust setting on your bread machine, and press start.
3. When the bread machine has finished baking, remove the bread and put it on a cooling rack.

Nutrition:

- Calories: 204
- Carbohydrates: 11 g
- Fat: 1 g
- Protein: 4 g
- Sodium: 480 mg

English muffin Bread

Preparation Time: 10 minutes
1 Pound Loaf

Ingredients:

- 1 teaspoon vinegar
- ¼ to 1/3 cup water
- 1 cup lukewarm milk
- 2 tablespoons butter or 2 tablespoons vegetable oil
- 1½ teaspoons salt
- 1½ teaspoons sugar
- ½ teaspoon baking powder
- 3½ cups unbleached all-purpose flour
- 2¼ teaspoons instant yeast

Directions:

1. Add each ingredient to the bread machine in the order and at the temperature recommended by your bread machine manufacturer.
2. Close the lid, select the basic bread, low crust setting on your bread machine, and press start.
3. When the bread machine has finished baking, remove the bread and put it on a cooling rack.

Nutrition:

- Calories: 190
- Carbohydrates: 13 g
- Fat: 1 g
- Protein: 2 g
- Sodium: 360 mg

Cranberry Orange Breakfast Bread

Preparation Time: 10 minutes
1½- Pound Loaf

Ingredients:

- 1½ cups orange juice
- 2 tablespoons vegetable oil
- 2 tablespoons honey
- 3 cups bread flour
- 1 tablespoon dry milk powder
- ½ teaspoon ground cinnamon
- ½ teaspoon ground allspice
- 1 teaspoon salt
- 1 (.25 ounce) package active dry yeast
- 1 tablespoon grated orange zest
- 1 cup sweetened dried cranberries
- 1/3 cup chopped walnuts

Directions:

1. Add each ingredient to the bread machine in the order and at the temperature recommended by your bread machine manufacturer.

2. Close the lid, select the basic bread, low crust setting on your bread machine, and press start.

3. Add the cranberries and chopped walnuts 5 to 5minutes before the last kneading cycle ends.

4. When the bread machine has finished baking, remove the bread and put it on a cooling rack.

Nutrition:

- Calories: 180
- Carbohydrates: 29 g
- Fat: 2 g
- Protein: 9 g
- Sodium: 249 mg

Buttermilk Honey Bread

Preparation Time: 10 minutes
1 Pound Loaf

Ingredients:

- ½ cup water
- ¾ cup buttermilk
- ¼ cup honey
- 3 tablespoons butter, softened and cut into pieces
- 3 cups bread flour
- 1½ teaspoons salt
- 2¼ teaspoons yeast (or 1 package)

Directions:

1. Add each ingredient to the bread machine in the order and at the temperature recommended by your bread machine manufacturer.
2. Close the lid, select the basic bread, medium crust setting on your bread machine, and press start.
3. When the bread machine has finished baking, remove the bread and put it on a cooling rack.

Nutrition:

- Calories: 224

- Carbohydrates: 19 g
- Fat: 1 g
- Protein: 2 g
- Sodium: 362 mg

Whole Wheat Breakfast Bread

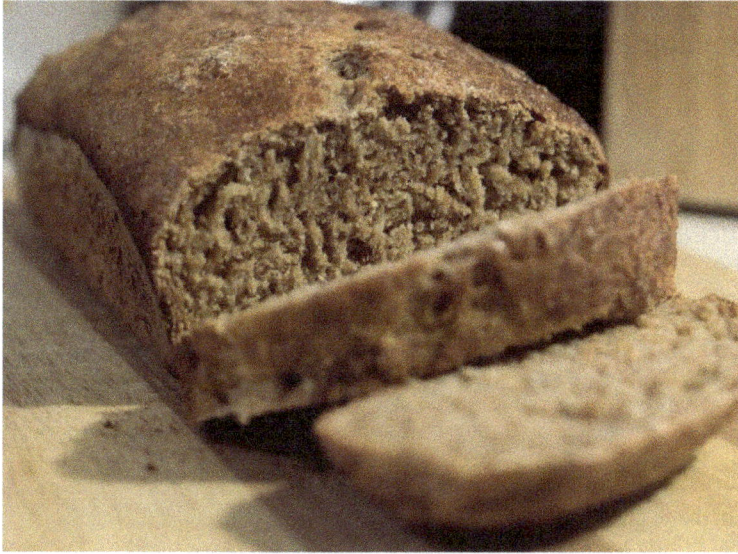

Preparation Time: 10 minutes

1½ -Pound Loaf

Ingredients:

- 3 cups white whole wheat flour
- ½ teaspoon salt
- 1 cup water
- ½ cup coconut oil, liquefied
- 4 tablespoons honey
- 2½ teaspoons active dry yeast

Directions:

1. Add each ingredient to the bread machine in the order and at the temperature recommended by your bread machine manufacturer.

2. Close the lid, select the basic bread, medium crust setting on your bread machine, and press start.

3. When the bread machine has finished baking, remove the bread and put it on a cooling rack.

Nutrition:

- Calories: 183
- Carbohydrates: 11 g
- Fat: 3 g
- Protein: 1 g
- Sodium: 120 mg

Cinnamon-Raisin Bread

Preparation Time: 25 minutes
1½-Pound Loaf

Ingredients:

- 1 cup water
- 2 tablespoons butter, softened
- 3 cups Gold Medal Better for Bread flour
- 3 tablespoons sugar
- 1½ teaspoons salt
- 1 teaspoon ground cinnamon
- 2½ teaspoons bread machine yeast
- ¾ cup raisins

Directions:

1. Add each ingredient except the raisins to the bread machine in the order and at the temperature recommended by your bread machine manufacturer.
2. Close the lid, select the sweet or basic bread, medium crust setting on your bread machine, and press start.
3. Add raisins 5minutes before the last kneading cycle ends.
4. When the bread machine has finished baking, remove the bread and put it on a cooling rack.

Nutrition:

- Calories: 181
- Carbohydrates: 31 g
- Fat: 2 g
- Protein: 4 g
- Sodium: 362 mg

Butter Bread Rolls

Preparation Time: 50 minutes

24 - Rolls

Ingredients:

- 1 cup warm milk
- ½ cup butter or ½ cup margarine, softened
- ¼ cup sugar
- 2 eggs
- 1½ teaspoons salt
- 4 cups bread flour
- 2¼ teaspoons active dry yeast

Directions:

1. In the bread machine pan, put all ingredients in the order suggested by the manufacturer.
2. Select dough setting.
3. When the cycle is completed, turn dough onto a lightly floured surface.
4. Divide dough into 24 portions.
5. Shape dough into balls.
6. Place in a greased 13 inch by the 9-inch baking pan.
7. Cover and let rise in a warm place for 30-45 minutes.
8. Bake at 350° F for 13-15minutes or until golden brown.

Nutrition:

- Calories: 211
- Carbohydrates: 31 g
- Fat: 2 g
- Protein: 4 g
- Sodium: 360 mg

Cranberry & Golden Raisin Bread

Preparation Time: 25 minutes

1½-Pound Loaf

Ingredients:

- 11/3 cups water
- 4 tablespoons sliced butter
- 3 cups flour
- 1 cup old fashioned oatmeal
- 1/3 cup brown sugar
- 1 teaspoon salt
- 4 tablespoons dried cranberries
- 4 tablespoons golden raisins
- 2 teaspoons bread machine yeast

Directions:

1. Add each ingredient except cranberries and golden raisins to the bread machine one by one, according to the manufacturer's instructions.

2. Close the lid, select the sweet or basic bread, medium crust setting on your bread machine, and press start.

3. Add the cranberries and golden raisins 5 to 5minutes before the last kneading cycle ends.

4. When the bread machine has finished baking, remove the bread and put it on a cooling rack.

Nutrition:

- Calories: 195
- Carbohydrates: 33 g
- Fat: 3 g
- Protein: 4 g
- Sodium: 240 mg

Breakfast Bread

Preparation Time: 55 minutes

1½-Pound Loaf

Ingredients:

- ½ teaspoon Xanthan gum
- ½ teaspoon salt
- 2 tablespoons coconut oil
- ½ cup butter, melted
- 1 teaspoon baking powder
- 2 cups of almond flour
- 7 eggs

Directions:

1. Preheat the oven to 355°F.
2. Beat eggs in a bowl on high for 2 minutes.
3. Add coconut oil and butter to the eggs and continue to beat.
4. Line a pan with baking paper and then pour the beaten eggs.
5. Pour in the rest of the ingredients and mix until it becomes thick.
6. Bake until a toothpick comes out dry. It takes 40 to 45 minutes.

Nutrition:

- Calories: 234
- Sodium: 122 mg
- Fat: 23g
- Carbohydrates: 10g
- Protein: 7g

Peanut Butter and Jelly Bread

Preparation Time: 10 minutes
1½-Pound Loaf

Ingredients:

- 1½ tablespoons vegetable oil
- 1 cup of water
- ½ cup blackberry jelly
- ½ cup peanut butter
- 1 teaspoon salt
- 1 tablespoon white sugar
- 2 cups of bread flour
- 1 cup whole-wheat flour
- 1½ teaspoons active dry yeast

Directions:

1. Put everything in your bread machine pan.
2. Select the basic setting.
3. Press the start button.
4. Take out the pan when done and set aside for 5minutes.

Nutrition:

- Calories: 193

- Carbohydrates: 11 g
- Fat: 9 g
- Cholesterol: 0 mg
- Protein: 4 g
- Fiber: 2 g
- Sugars: 11 g
- Sodium: 244 mg
- Potassium: 1 mg

Low-Carb Bagel

Preparation Time: 1 hour
1½-Pound Loaf

Ingredients:

- 1 cup protein powder, unflavored
- 1/3 cup coconut flour
- 1 teaspoon baking powder
- ½ teaspoon sea salt
- ¼ cup ground flaxseed
- 1/3 cup sour cream
- 1½ eggs

Seasoning topping:

- 1 teaspoon dried parsley
- 1 teaspoon dried oregano
- 1 teaspoon dried minced onion
- ½ teaspoon garlic powder
- ½ teaspoon dried basil
- ½ teaspoon sea salt

Directions:

1. Preheat the oven to 350° F.

2. In a mixer, blend sour cream and eggs until well combined.

3. Whisk together the flaxseed, salt, baking powder, Protein: powder, and coconut flour in a bowl.

4. Mix the dry ingredients until it becomes wet ingredients. Make sure it is well blended.

5. Whisk the topping seasoning together in a small bowl. Set aside.

6. Grease 2 donut pans that can contain six donuts each.

7. Sprinkle pan with about 1 teaspoon. Topping seasoning and evenly pour batter into each.

8. Sprinkle the top of each bagel evenly with the rest of the seasoning mixture.

9. Bake in the oven for 25 minutes, or until golden brown.

Nutrition:

- Calories: 174
- Sodium: 267 mg
- Fat: 6.1 g
- Carbohydrates: 4.2 g
- Protein: 1½ g

Puri Bread

Preparation Time: 1 hour
1-Pound Loaf

Ingredients:
- 1 cup almond flour, sifted
- ½ cup of warm water
- 2 tablespoons clarified butter
- 1 cup olive oil for frying
- Salt to taste

Directions:
1. Salt the water and add the flour.
2. Make some holes in the center of the dough and pour warm clarified butter.
3. Knead the dough and let stand for 15 minutes, covered.
4. Shape into six balls.
5. Flatten the balls into six thin rounds using a rolling pin.
6. Heat enough oil to cover a round frying pan completely.
7. Place a puri in it when hot.
8. Fry for 1 second on each side.
9. Place on a paper towel.
10. Repeat with the rest of the puri and serve.

Nutrition:

- Calories: 176
- Fat: 3 g
- Carbohydrates: 6 g
- Protein: 3 g
- Sodium: 80 mg

Bread Roll

Preparation Time: 1 hour
1-Pound Loaf

Ingredients:

- 2 tablespoons coconut oil, melted
- 6 tablespoons coconut flour
- ¼ teaspoon baking soda
- 1 tablespoon Italian seasoning
- ½ teaspoon salt
- 2 tablespoons gelatin
- 6 tablespoons hot water

Directions:

1. Preheat the oven to 300° F (150°C).

2. Mix the coconut oil, coconut flour, and baking soda.

3. In a separate bowl, whisk together the gelatin and hot water to create your gelatin egg.

4. Pour the gelatin egg into the coconut flour mixture and combine well.

5. Add in the Italian seasoning and salt to taste (you can taste the mixture to see if you want to add more) and mix well into a dough.

6. Use your hands to form 2 small rolls from the dough, place the rolls on a baking tray lined with parchment

paper, and bake in the oven for 40-50 minutes until the outside of each roll is lightly browned and crispy like you'd typically find in a regular breadroll.

7. Let the rolls cool down before serving so that the gelatin sets a bit and can hold the roll together. Enjoy at room temperature with some ghee or coconutoil.

8. This recipe can be doubled, tripled, etc. If you want to make more AIP bread rolls at the sametime.

Nutrition:

- Calories: 290
- Sodium: 320 mg
- Fat: 23.6 g
- Carbohydrates: 11 g
- Protein: 33.5 g

Bacon Breakfast Bagels

Preparation Time: 2 hours

2-PoundLoaf

Ingredients:

- Bagels
- ¾ cup (61 g) almond flour
- 1 teaspoon Xanthan gum
- 1 large egg
- 1½ cups grated mozzarella
- 2 tablespoons cream cheese
- toppings
- 1 tablespoon butter, melted
- 1 teaspoon salt
- Sesame seeds to taste
- fillings
- 2 tablespoons pesto
- 2 tablespoons cream cheese
- 1 cup arugula leaves
- 6 slices grilled streaky bacon

Directions:

1. Preheat oven to 390° F.

2. In a bowl mix together the almond flour and Xanthan gum. Then add the egg and mix together until well combined. Set a side. It will look like a doughy ball.

3. In a pot over a medium-low heat slowly melt the creamcheese and mozzarella together and remove from heat once melted. This can be done in the microwave as well.

4. Add your melted cheese mix to the almond flour mix and knead until well combined. The Mozzarella mix will stick together in a bit of a ball but don't worry, persist with it. It will all combine well eventually. It's important to get the Xanthan gum incorporated through the cheese mix. Suppose the dough gets too tough to work, place in microwave for few seconds to warm and repeat until you have some thing that resembles a dough.

5. Split your dough into 3 pieces and roll into round logs. If you have a donut pan, place yourlogs into the pan. If not, make circles with each logand join together and place on a baking tray. Try to make sure you have nice little circles. The other way to do this is to make a ball and flattens lightly on the baking tray and cut a circle out of the middle if you have a small cookie cutter.

6. Melt your butter and brush over the top of your bagels and sprinkle sesame seeds or your topping of choice. The butter should help the seeds stick. Garlic and onion powder or cheesemake nice additions if you have them for savory bagels.

7. Place bagels in the oven for about 11½ minutes. Keep an eye on them. The topsshouldgo golden brown.

8. Take the bagels out of the oven and allow to cool.

9. If you like your bagels toasted, cut them in half lengthwise and place back in the oven until slightly golden and toasty.

10. Spread bagel with cream chease, cover in pesto, add a few arugula leaves and top with your crispybacon (or your filling of choice.)

Nutrition:

- Calories: 605
- Fat: 50 g
- Carbohydrates: 57 g
- Protein: 30.1 g
- Sodium: 295 mg

Hot Dog Buns

Preparation Time: 1 hour

1-Pound Loaf

Ingredients:

- 1¼ cups almond flour
- 5 tablespoons psyllium husk powder
- 1 teaspoon sea salt
- 2 teaspoons baking powder
- 1¼ cups boiling water
- 2 teaspoons lemon juice
- 3 eggs whites

Directions:

1. Preheat the oven to 350° F
2. In a bowl, put all dry ingredients and mix well.
3. Add boiling water, lemon juice, and egg whites into the dry mixture and whisk until combined.
4. Mould the dough into ten portions and roll into buns.
5. Transfer into the preheated oven and cook for 40 to 50 minutes on the lower oven rack.
6. Check for doneness and remove it.
7. Top with desired toppings and hot dogs.
8. Serve.

Nutrition:

- Calories: 214
- Fat: 1½ g
- Carbohydrates: 4 g
- Protein: 4 g
- Sodium: 242 mg

Paleo Coconut Bread

Preparation Time: 1 hour

1½ -Pound Loaf

Ingredients:

- ½ cup coconut flour
- ¼ cup almond milk (unsweetened)
- ¼ cup coconut oil (melted)
- 6 eggs
- ¼ teaspoon baking soda
- ¼ teaspoon salt

Directions:

1. Preheat the oven to 350° F.
2. Prepare a (1½ x 4) bread pan with parchment paper.
3. In a bowl, combine salt, baking soda, and coconut flour.
4. Combine the oil, milk, and eggs in another bowl.
5. Gradually add the wet ingredients into the dry ingredients and mix well.
6. Pour the mixture into the prepared pan.
7. Bake for 40 to 50 minutes.
8. Cool, slice, and serve.

Nutrition:

- Calories: 191
- Fat: 11 g
- Carbohydrates: 3.4 g
- Protein: 4.2 g
- Sodium: 220 mg

Healthy Low Carb Bread

Preparation Time: 1 hour

1½-Pound Loaf

Ingredients:

- 2/3 cup coconut flour
- 2/3 cup coconut oil (softened not melted)
- 9 eggs
- 2 teaspoons cream of tartar
- ¾ teaspoon Xanthan gum
- 1 teaspoon baking soda
- ¼ teaspoon salt

Directions:

1. Preheat the oven to 350° F.
2. Grease a pound pan with 1 to 2 teaspoons. Melted coconut oil and place it in the freezer to harden.
3. Add eggs into a bowl and mix for 2 minutes with a hand mixer.
4. Add coconut oil into the eggs and mix.
5. Add dry ingredients to a second bowl and whisk until mixed.
6. Put the dry ingredients into the egg mixture and mix on low speed with a hand mixer until dough is formed and the mixture is incorporated.

7. Add the dough into the prepared pound pan, transfer it into the preheated oven, and bake for 35 minutes.

8. Take out the bread pan from the oven.

9. Cool, slice, and serve.

Nutrition:

- Calories: 229
- Carbohydrates: 6 g
- Sodium: 60 mg
- Fat: 25.5 g
- Protein: 4 g

Spicy Bread

Preparation Time: 1 hour

1½-Pound Loaf

Ingredients:

- ½ cup coconut flour
- 6 eggs
- 3 large jalapenos, sliced
- 4 ounces' turkey bacon, sliced
- ½ cup ghee
- ¼ teaspoon baking soda
- ¼ teaspoon salt
- ¼ cup of water

Directions:

1. Preheat the oven to 400°F.
2. Cut bacon and jalapenos on a baking tray and roast for 1 1/4 minutes.
3. Flip and bake for five more minutes.
4. Remove seeds from the jalapenos.
5. Place jalapenos and bacon pounds in a food processor and blend until smooth.
6. In a bowl, add ghee, eggs, and ¼-cup water. Mix well.

7. Then add some coconut flour, baking soda, and salt. Stir to mix.

8. Add bacon and jalapeno mix.

9. Grease the pound pan with ghee.

10. Pour batter into the pound pan.

11. Bake for 40 minutes.

12. Enjoy.

Nutrition:

- Calories: 240
- Sodium: 180 mg
- Carbohydrates: 7 g
- Fat: 1g

Fluffy Paleo Bread

Preparation Time: 1 hour
2-Pound Loaf

Ingredients:

- 1¼ cups almond flour
- 5 eggs
- 1 teaspoon lemon juice
- 1/3 cup avocado oil
- 1 dash black pepper
- ½ teaspoon sea salt
- 3 to 4 tablespoons tapioca flour
- 1 to 2 teaspoons poppy seed
- ¼ cup ground flaxseed
- ½ teaspoon baking soda
- top with:
- poppy seeds
- pumpkin seeds

Directions:

1. Preheat the oven to 350° F.
2. Line a baking pan with parchment paper and set aside.

3. In a bowl, add eggs, avocado oil, and lemon juice and whisk until combined.

4. In another bowl, add tapioca flour, almond flour, baking soda, flaxseed, black pepper, and poppy seed. Mix.

5. Add the lemon juice mixture into the flour mixture and mix well.

6. Add the batter into the prepared pound pan and top with extra pumpkin seeds and poppy seeds.

7. Cover pound pan and transfer into the prepared oven, and bake for 1 minute. Remove cover and bake until an inserted knife comes out clean after about 15 minutes.

8. Remove from oven and cool.

9. Slice and serve.

Nutrition:

- Calories: 190
- Sodium: 190 mg
- Fat: 2 g
- Carbohydrates: 4.4 g

German Pumpernickel Bread

Preparation Time: 10 minutes
2-Pound Loaf

Ingredients:

- 1½ tablespoons vegetable oil
- 1½ cups warm water
- 3 tablespoons cocoa
- 1/3 cup molasses
- 1½ teaspoons salt
- 1 tablespoon caraway seeds
- 1 cup rye flour
- 1½ cups of bread flour
- 1½ tablespoons wheat gluten
- 1 cup whole wheat flour
- 2½ teaspoons bread machine yeast

Directions:

1. Put everything in your bread machine.
2. Select the primary cycle.
3. Hit the start button.
4. Transfer bread to a rack for cooling once done.

Nutrition:

- Calories: 189
- Carbohydrates: 22.4 g
- Total Fat 2.3 g
- Cholesterol: 0mg
- Protein: 3 g
- Sodium: 360 mg

European Black Bread

Preparation Time: 10 minutes
1½-Pound Loaf

Ingredients:

- 1 cup of water
- ¾ teaspoon cider vinegar
- ½ cup rye flour
- 1½ cups flour
- 1 tablespoon margarine
- ¼ cup of oat bran
- 1 teaspoon salt
- 1½ tablespoons sugar
- 1 teaspoon dried onion flakes
- 1 teaspoon caraway seed
- 1 teaspoon yeast
- 2 tablespoons unsweetened cocoa

Directions:

1. Put everything in your bread machine.
2. Now select the basic setting.
3. Hit the start button.
4. Transfer bread to a rack for cooling once done.

Nutrition:

- Calories: 191
- Carbohydrates: 22 g
- Total fat: 1.7 g
- Cholesterol: 0mg
- Protein: 3 g
- Sugar: 2 g
- Sodium: 247 mg

French Baguettes

Preparation Time: 25 minutes
1½-Pound Loaf

Ingredients:

- 1¼ cups warm water
- 3½ cups bread flour
- 1 teaspoon salt
- 1 package active dry yeast

Directions:

1. Place ingredients in the bread machine. Select the dough cycle. Hit the start button.
2. When the dough cycle is finished, remove it with floured hands and cut in half on a well-floured.
3. Take each half of the dough and roll it to make a pound about 1½ inches long in the shape of French bread.
4. Place on a greased baking sheet and cover with a towel.
5. Let rise until doubled, about 1 hour.
6. Preheat oven to 450° F (210° C).
7. Bake until golden brown, turning the pan around once halfway during baking.
8. Transfer the loaves to a rack.

Nutrition:

- Calories: 161
- Carbohydrates: 42 g
- Total Fat 0.6 g
- Cholesterol: 0 mg
- Protein: 6 g
- Fiber: 1.7 g
- Sugars: 0.1 g
- Sodium: 240 mg

Portuguese Sweet Bread

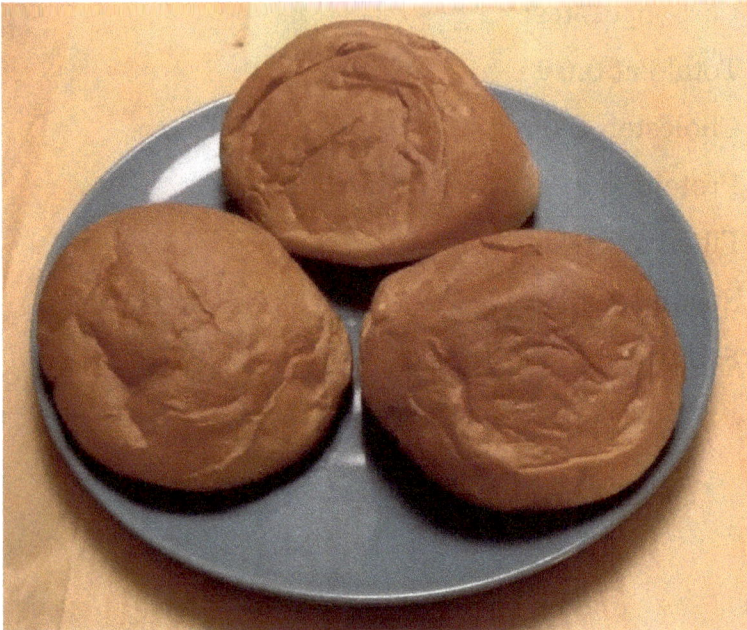

Preparation Time: 10 minutes

1-Pound Loaf

Ingredients:

- 1 egg beaten
- 1 cup milk
- 1/3 cup sugar
- 2 tablespoons margarine
- 3 cups bread flour
- ¾ teaspoon salt

- 2½ teaspoons active dry yeast

Directions:

1. Place everything into your bread machine.
2. Select the sweet bread setting. Hit the start button.
3. Transfer the loaves to a rack for cooling once done.

Nutrition:

- Calories: 179
- Carbohydrates: 24 g
- Total Fat: 11½ g
- Cholesterol: 1 mg
- Protein: 3 g
- Fiber: 0g
- Sugars: 4 g
- Sodium: 180 mg

Italian Bread

Preparation Time: 2 hours
1-Pound Loaf

Ingredients:

- 1 tablespoon of light brown sugar
- 4 cups all-purpose flour, unbleached
- 1½ teaspoons of salt
- 11/3 cups + 1 tablespoon warm water
- 1 package active dry yeast
- 1½ teaspoons of olive oil
- 1 egg
- 2 tablespoons cornmeal

Directions:

1. Place flour, brown sugar, 1/3 cup warm water, salt, olive oil, and yeast in your bread machine. Select the dough cycle. Hit the start button.
2. Deflate your dough. Turn it on a floured surface.
3. Form two loaves from the dough.
4. Keep them on your cutting board. The seam side should be down. Sprinkle some cornmeal on your board.
5. Place a damp cloth on your loaves to cover them.
6. Wait for 40 minutes. The volume should double.

7. In the meantime, preheat your oven to 190° C.

8. Beat 1 tablespoon of water and an egg in a bowl.

9. Brush this mixture on your loaves.

10. Make an extended cut at the center of your loaves with a knife.

11. Shake your cutting board gently, making sure that the loaves do not stick.

12. Now slide your loaves on a baking sheet.

13. Bake in your oven for about 35 minutes.

Nutrition:

- Calories: 165
- Carbohydrates: 1.6 g
- Total Fat: 0.9 g
- Cholesterol: 9 mg
- Protein: 3.1 g
- Fiber: 1 g
- Sugars: 1g
- Sodium: 360 mg
- Potassium: 39 mg

Pita Bread

Preparation Time: 1 hour

1½-PoundLoaf

Ingredients:

- 3 cups of all-purpose flour
- 1½ cups warm water
- 1 tablespoon of vegetable oil
- 1 teaspoon salt
- 1½ teaspoons active dry yeast
- 1 active teaspoon white sugar

Directions:

1. Place all the ingredients in your bread pan.
2. Select the dough setting. Hit the start button.
3. The machine beeps after the dough rises adequately.
4. Turn the dough on a floured surface.
5. Roll and stretch the dough gently into a 1½ inch rope.
6. Cut into eight pieces with a knife.
7. Now roll each piece into a ball. It should be smooth.
8. Roll each ball into a 7-inch circle. Keep covered with a towel on a floured top for 30 minutes for the pita to rise. It should get puffy slightly.
9. Preheat your oven to 260° C.

10. Keep the pitas on your wire cake rack. Transfer to the oven rack directly.

11. Bake the pitas for 5 minutes. They should be puffed. The top should start to brown.

12. Take out from the oven. Keep the pitas immediately in a sealed paper bag. You can also cover using a damp kitchen towel.

13. Split the top edge or cut it into half once the pitas are soft. You can also have the whole pitas if you want.

Nutrition:

- Calories: 191
- Carbohydrates: 37 g
- Total Fat: 3g
- Cholesterol: 0mg
- Protein: 5g
- Fiber: 1g
- Sugars: 1g
- Sodium: 243mg
- Potassium: 66mg

Syrian Bread

Preparation Time: 1 hour

1½-Pound Loaf

Ingredients:

- 2 tablespoons vegetable oil
- 1 cup of water
- 1½ teaspoon salt
- ½ teaspoon white sugar
- 1½ teaspoons active dry yeast
- 3 cups all-purpose flour

Directions:

1. Put everything in your bread machine pan.
2. Select the dough cycle. Hit the start button.
3. Preheat your oven to 475 degrees F.
4. Turn to dough on a lightly floured surface once done.
5. Divide it into eight equal pieces. Form them into rounds.
6. Take a damp cloth and cover the rounds with it.
7. Now roll the dough into flat thin circles. They should have a diameter of around 1½ inches.
8. Cook in your preheated baking sheets until they are golden brown and puffed.

Nutrition:

- Calories: 169
- Carbohydrates: 36 g
- Total Fat 5 g
- Protein: 5 g
- Fiber: 1 g
- Sugar: 0 g
- Sodium: 360 mg
- Potassium: 66 mg

Ethiopian Milk and Honey Bread

Preparation Time: 10 minutes

1-Pound Loaf

Ingredients:

- 3 tablespoons honey
- 1 cup + 1 tablespoon milk
- 3 cups bread flour
- 3 tablespoons melted butter
- 2 teaspoons active dry yeast
- 1½ teaspoon salt

Directions:

1. Add everything to the pan of your bread
2. Select the white bread or basic setting and the medium crust setting.
3. Hit the start button.
4. Take out your hot pound once it is done.
5. Keep on your wire rack for cooling.
6. Slice your bread once it is cold and serve.

Nutrition:

- Calories: 189
- Carbohydrates: 1 g
- Total Fat 3.1 g
- Cholesterol: 0 mg
- Protein: 2.4 g
- Fiber: 0.6 g
- Sugars: 3.3 g
- Sodium: 362 mg

Swedish Cardamom Bread

Preparation Time: 1 hour

1-Pound Loaf

Ingredients:

- ¼ cup of sugar
- ¾ cup of warm milk
- ¾ teaspoon cardamom
- ½ teaspoon salt
- ¼ cup of softened butter
- 1 egg
- 2¼ teaspoons bread machine yeast
- 3 cups all-purpose flour
- 5 tablespoons milk for brushing
- 2 tablespoons sugar for sprinkling

Directions:

1. Put everything (except milk for brushing and sugar for sprinkling) in the pan of your bread machine.
2. Select the dough cycle. Hit the start button. You should have an elastic and smooth dough once the process is complete. It should be double in size.
3. Transfer to a lightly floured surface.
4. Now divide into three balls. Set aside for 5minutes.

5. Roll all the balls into long ropes of around 1 inch.

6. Braid the shapes. Pinch ends under securely and keeps on a cookie sheet. You can also divide your dough into two balls. Smooth them and keep them on your bread pan.

7. Brush milk over the braid. Sprinkle sugar lightly.

8. Now bake in your oven for 25 minutes at 375° F (190° C).

9. Take a foil and cover for the final 5minutes. It's prevents over-browning.

10. Transfer to your cooling rack.

Nutrition:

- Calories: 185
- Carbohydrates: 22 g
- Total Fat: 7g
- Cholesterol: 1mg
- Protein: 3g
- Fiber: 1 g
- Sugars: 3g
- Sodium: 145 mg

Fiji Sweet Potato Bread

Preparation Time: 10 minutes
1-Pound Loaf

Ingredients:

- 1 teaspoon vanilla extract
- ½ cup of warm water
- 4 cups flour
- 1 cup sweet mashed potatoes
- 2 tablespoons softened butter
- ½ teaspoon cinnamon
- 1½ teaspoons salt
- 1/3 cup brown sugar
- 2 tablespoons powdered milk
- 2 teaspoons yeast

Directions:

1. Add everything in the pan of your bread.
2. Select the white bread and the crust you want.
3. Hit the start button.
4. Set aside on wire racks for cooling before slicing.

Nutrition:

- Calories: 182
- Carbohydrates: 21 g
- Fat: 5 g
- Protein: 4 g
- Fiber: 1 g
- Sugar 3 g
- Sodium: 360 mg

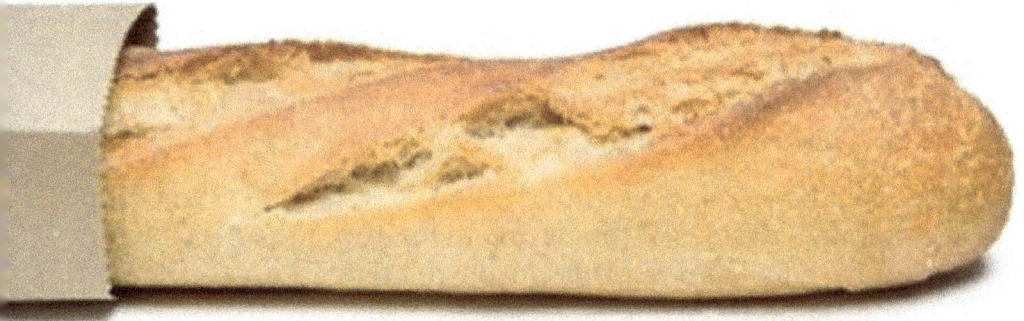

Sourdough Baguette

Preparation Time: 1 hour

2 -Pound Loaf

Ingredients:

- 3¼ cups bread flour
- 1 cup sourdough starter
- 1 cup water
- 1¾ teaspoons fine sea salt

Directions:

1. Mix the starter, flour, water, and salt. Mix with a spatula until you get a shaggy dough. Cover using a kitchen towel and leave for 30 minutes.

2. Knead for 5minutes until the dough starts to feel smooth. Scrape the sides of the bowl and lightly oil the insides. Form a ball and put it in the bowl. Cover again and leave for 2-4 hours to double in size.

3. Punch the dough down on a floured surface. Make a rectangle from the dough and fold it in thirds to the middle beginning from one short side. Pinch the ends closed. Put the dough back into the bowl, cover, and leave for 30 minutes. Repeat this step again.

4. Divide your dough evenly into 3 pieces.

5. Put them on a floured work surface to form baguettes. Line a rimless baking sheet with a piece of parchment

paper and transfer the baguettes onto it. Cover with a kitchen towel and leave for 30 minutes.

6. Meanwhile, preheat the oven to 450°F. Put a baking sheet on the middle rack and a cast-iron skillet on the rack below. Prepare a cup of ice cubes.

7. When baguettes have almost doubled in size, cut few slashes on their tops with a knife. Lightly dampen them and place them on the hot baking sheet. Pour the ice cubes into the skillet and close the oven door. Set to 400° F and bake for 1 minute. Bake for longer if you want your crust deep colored.

8. Take them out and let them cool for 30 minutes before slicing.

Nutrition:

- Calories: 175

- Carbohydrates: 24 g

- Fat: 0 g

- Protein:2 g

- Sodium: 360 g

Classic French Baguette

Preparation Time: 30 min. + 11 hours

2-Pound Loaf

Ingredients:

For the poolish:

- ¾ cup bread flour
- 6 tablespoons + 1 teaspoon filtered water, warm 90°F
- ¼ teaspoon active dry yeast

For the final dough:

- 1¾ cups bread flour
- ½ cup all-purpose flour
- ½ cup + 3 tablespoons filtered water, warm 90°F
- ¼ teaspoon active dry yeast
- 1¼ teaspoon kosher salt

Directions:

1. Make a poolish in advance. Mix all of the ingredients in a large bowl. Cover it with plastic wrap and leave for 1½ – 5hours.

2. Then, add all of the ingredients for the dough to the poolish. Stir well to combine. Knead it with your hands until you get a shaggy dough and leave for 30 minutes covered with plastic wrap.

3. Next, dampen your hands and pull on and stretch up one side of the dough, then fold down over the top of the dough. Repeat for each side after the rotating bowl 90 degrees when the last side is done. Cover and leave for 30 minutes. Repeat this process four times.

4. Meanwhile, prepare the equipment: set one oven rack in the middle and another at the bottom position. Put an upside-down sheet pan on the middle rack. Preheat the oven to 500° F for 1 hour. Flour a lint-free towel and line an undimmed baking sheet with parchment paper.

5. Divide the dough into two equal portions by cutting it. Place them on a lightly floured surface. Form a rectangle from one piece of dough and carefully stretch out the short ends. Fold every short end to the center, press it down with your fingertips to seal. Do the same with every long end to create a seam in the dough. Repeat this process with another piece. Cover both pieces with plastic wrap and leave for 5minutes.

6. Place one-piece seam side up and press it into a thin rectangle. Start folding down your dough (½") and sealing it with fingerprints, beginning from the top-left edge. Work across the top in the same way. Create a tight log by continuing folding down on the dough and sealing it. You should get a thin, tight log. Flip it seam side down. Roll your dough evenly into a long thin snake shape using both hands. Work it into a 1" baguette. Transfer it onto the prepared floured towel. Create the folds for holding the dough's shape by pushing a towel up on both sides of the baguette. Repeat all the steps for the second portion. Cover the baguettes with plastic wrap and leave for 1 hour to rise.

7. Carefully flip the baguettes onto parchment paper, seam side down. Cut 4-5 ¼" deep diagonal slashes on the top of the baguettes with a sharp knife.

8. Prepare a small bowl filled with 2 cups of ice cubes. Open the oven and gently slide the whole piece of parchment paper with the baguettes onto the preheated sheet pan. Pour ice into the preheated skillet and close the oven door immediately. Turn the temperature down to 475° F and bake for about 25-40 minutes depending on what crust you want for your baguettes.

9. Take them out of the oven and transfer them to a cooling rack. Let them cool for 30 minutes before slicing.

Nutrition:

- Calories: 172
- Carbohydrates:15 g
- Fat: 0 g
- Protein: 3 g
- Sodium: 360 mg

Alternative French Baguettes

Preparation Time: 10 minutes +2 h.

1½ -Pound Loaf

Ingredients:

- olive oil, for greasing
- 3¾ cups strong white bread flour, plus extra for dusting
- 2 teaspoons salt
- 2 teaspoons fast-action yeast
- 1½ cups cool water

Directions:

1. Oil a 2¼ liter square plastic container with olive oil.

2. Prepare a freestanding mixer with a dough hook and add salt, flour, and yeast to its bowl. Pour in the water (three-quarters) and start mixing at a slow speed. Gradually pour in the rest of the water when the dough comes together and mix for 5-7 minutes at a medium speed. You should get an elastic and glossy dough.

3. Transfer the dough to the oiled container, cover, and leave for 1 hour.

4. Dust a linen baker couche and the work surface with flour. Gently place your dough onto the work surface.

5. Divide it evenly into 4 portions. Flatten the dough and fold its sides to the center to form an oblong from each piece. Roll every piece up into a sausage with a smooth

top and join through the whole length of the base. Starting from the middle, roll each piece with both hands. Make a forward and backward movement without heavy pressing to roll out 1½" long baguettes.

6. Place a baguette along the edge of the couche and pleat it up against the edge of the bread. Repeat for all of the baguettes—they should be lined up against each other and divided with a pleat between each. Cover with a tea towel and leave for 1 hour to double in size.

7. Preheat the oven to 465° F and put a roasting tray in the bottom.

8. When the dough has doubled in size, put them on the work surface, and dust it with flour. Make four slashes along the length of the baguette with a sharp knife. Place each baguette on a baking tray.

9. Put the bread into the oven and pour the hot water on the roasting tray for steam. Close the oven and bake for 10-20 minutes or longer for a deep color.

10. Take out of the oven and let the baguettes cool completely before slicing.

Nutrition:

- Calories: 170
- Carbohydrates:18 g
- Fat:0 g
- Protein:3 g
- Sodium: 480 mg

Whole-Wheat Baguette

Preparation Time: 2 h 40 min.

2 -Pound Loaf

Ingredients:

- 3 cups warm water 80°F
- 1½ tablespoons granulated yeast
- 1½ tablespoons kosher salt
- 2½ cups ground hard white wheat flour
- 4 cups all-purpose flour

Directions:

1. Mix the yeast, water, and salt in a large bowl. Combine the flours in another bowl and mix well. Add the mixed flour to a bowl with water and stir with a wooden spoon. Knead with your hands if it's hard to stir. Cover with plastic wrap and leave for 4-5 hours until it begins to flatten on top.

2. Preheat the oven to 450° F. Place a baking stone on the central oven rack and a cast-iron skillet on a lower shelf.

3. Dust the dough top with flour and cut off a 1lb portion. Return the rested dough to the fridge.

4. Dust your dough lightly with flour and form into a ball. When it's cohesive, stretch and elongate it to create a cylinder (2" in diameter). Dust a piece of the parchment with whole wheat flour. Transfer the pound onto the paper and leave for 1 minute.

5. Next, lightly dampen the surface of the pound. Make a few diagonal slashes across the top of the baguette with a serrated bread knife.

6. Transfer it onto the hot stone and pour 1 cup of hot water into the skillet. Close the oven and bake for 25 minutes or longer to get the deep brown crust.

7. Remove and let it cool for 40 minutes before slicing.

Nutrition:

- Carbohydrates: 5 g

- Fat: 00 g

- Protein: 2 g

- Calories: 169

- Sodium: 360 mg

Gluten-Free French Baguette

Preparation Time: 10 min. + 1 h.
1- Pound Loaf

Ingredients:

- 1 cup gluten-free white rice flour
- ½ cup arrowroot flour
- 1½ teaspoons Xanthan gum
- ¾ teaspoon Himalayan fine salt
- ¾ cup warm water
- 1 tablespoon pure maple syrup
- 2 ¼ teaspoons gluten-free active dry yeast
- 1 tablespoon extra virgin olive oil + some for brushing
- 2 large egg whites, at room temperature, whisked
- ½ teaspoon apple cider vinegar

Directions:

1. Mix all of the dry ingredients in a large bowl.
2. Mix the water, maple syrup, and yeast in another bowl. Leave it for 5minutes until the yeast foams.
3. Add the olive oil, yeast, egg whites, and vinegar to the dry mixture. Beat for 1 minute with a mixer. Scrape the sides while mixing.

4. Put your dough onto a greased French bread pan and spoon with olive oil. Make a few slashes diagonally and brush with olive oil. Cover tightly with a kitchen towel and leave for 40 minutes in a warm place.

5. Preheat the oven to 400°F and transfer the dough into it. Bake for 35-40 minutes until it has a nice golden crust.

6. Take out from the oven and let it cool for 40 minutes before slicing.

Nutrition:

- Calories: 181
- Carbohydrates: 15 g
- Fat: 2 g
- Protein: 2 g
- Sodium: 170 mg

www.ingramcontent.com/pod-product-compliance
Lightning Source LLC
Chambersburg PA
CBHW050747030426
42336CB00012B/1705